WHY WE SLEEP COOKBOOK

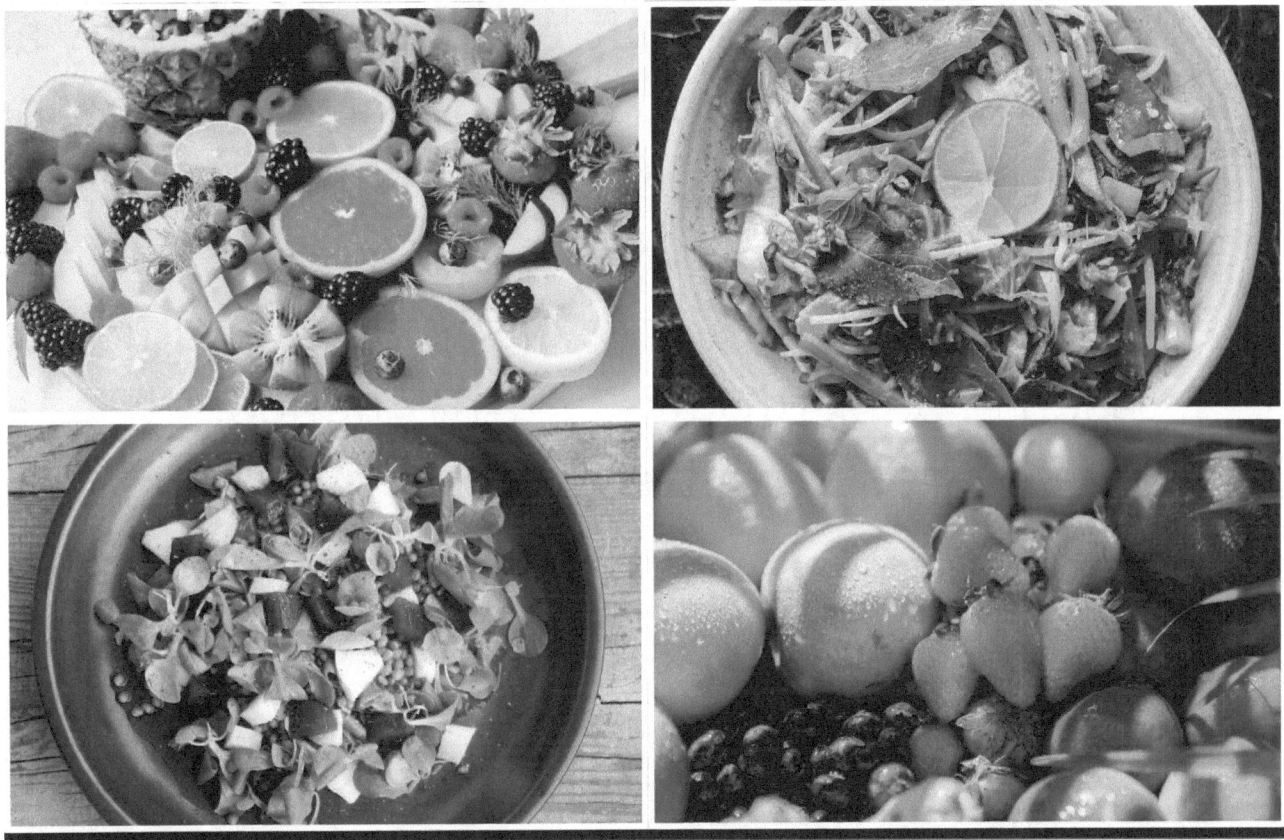

300 Transforming Recipes Inspired by Matthew Walker for Unlocking the Secrets of Restful Nights Through Nourishing Meals

Charlene Soluri

Copyright © 2025 Charlene Soluri

All rights reserved.

No part of this publication may be reproduced, distributed, or transmitted in any form or by any means, including photocopying, recording, or other electronic or mechanical methods, without the prior written permission of the publisher, except in the case of brief quotations used in book reviews or other noncommercial uses permitted by copyright law

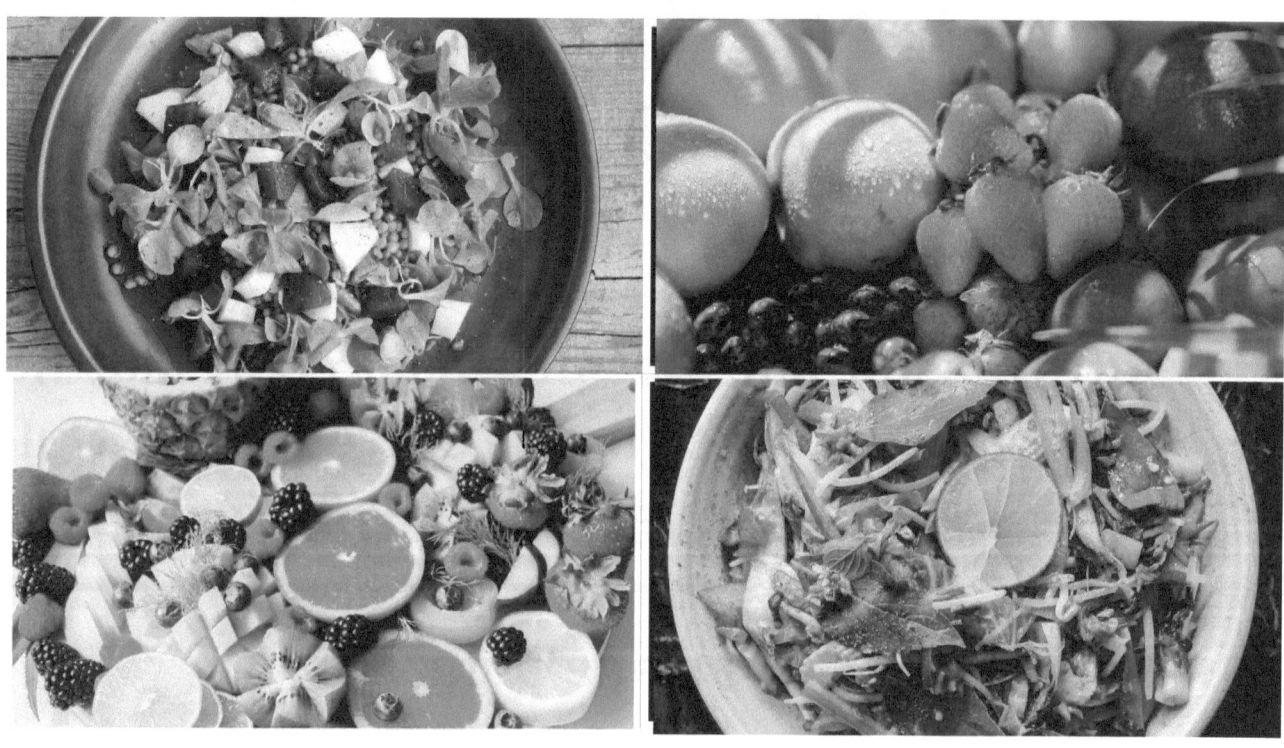

Table of Contents

Introduction..7
The Connection Between Sleep and Nutrition..8
   How Food Impacts Sleep Quality..8
   The Science of Sleep-Friendly Nutrients..10
   Creating an Evening Ritual with Food..11
Meal Planning for Sleep Optimization...13
   Weekly Sleep-Friendly Meal Plans..14
   Tips for Structuring Evening Meals..16
   Foods to Avoid Before Bed..17
Lifestyle Practices for Better Sleep...18
   Combining Nutrition with Sleep Hygiene Practices.....................................19
   Meditation and Relaxation Techniques After Dinner..................................20
   Ideal Meal Timing for Optimal Sleep..21
Morning Meals for Balanced Sleep..22
   Banana and Almond Butter Oatmeal..22
   Greek Yogurt with Berries and Walnuts..23
   Spinach and Feta Omelette...24
   Avocado Toast with Whole Grain Bread..25
   Smoothie with Cherries, Spinach, and Almond Milk....................................26
   Quinoa Breakfast Bowl with Nuts and Fruits..27
   Whole Wheat Pancakes with Banana and Honey...28
   Cottage Cheese and Pineapple Bowl..29
   Scrambled Eggs with Smoked Salmon and Arugula....................................30
   Tofu and Veggie Breakfast Wrap..31
Energizing Lunches Without Disrupting Sleep..32
   Grilled Chicken and Quinoa Salad..32
   Lentil and Vegetable Stew..33
   Turkey and Avocado Wrap...34
   Chickpea and Spinach Stir-Fry...35
   Salmon and Brown Rice Bowl..36

    Hummus and Vegetable Pita 37

    Grilled Veggie and Goat Cheese Sandwich 38

    Shrimp and Avocado Salad 39

    Sweet Potato and Black Bean Bowl 40

    Chicken and Vegetable Stir-Fry 41

Sleep-Promoting Dinners 42

    Grilled Salmon with Quinoa and Asparagus 42

    Turkey and Sweet Potato Bowl 43

    Tofu and Vegetable Stir-Fry 44

    Chicken and Brown Rice with Kale 45

    Lentil and Vegetable Stew 46

    Shrimp and Avocado Salad 47

    Cod with Lemon and Steamed Veggies 48

    Chickpea and Spinach Curry 49

    Baked Chicken with Sweet Potato and Green Beans 50

    Quinoa-Stuffed Bell Peppers 51

Soothing Snacks for a Restful Night 52

    Banana and Almond Butter Bites 52

    Greek Yogurt with Honey and Walnuts 53

    Chamomile Tea with Whole-Grain Crackers and Cheese 54

    Kiwi and Pumpkin Seeds Bowl 55

    Warm Oatmeal with Cinnamon and Almonds 56

    Apple Slices with Peanut Butter 57

    Cottage Cheese with Pineapple 58

    Avocado Toast on Whole-Grain Bread 59

    Herbal Tea with Dark Chocolate 60

    Warm Milk with Nutmeg 61

Calming Teas and Smoothies 62

    Chamomile Lavender Tea 62

    Banana Almond Sleep Smoothie 63

    Valerian Root Tea 64

    Kiwi and Spinach Sleep Smoothie 65

    Peppermint Herbal Tea 66

    Tart Cherry and Almond Smoothie 67

    Lemon Balm Tea 68

    Golden Milk Smoothie 69

    Ashwagandha Sleep Smoothie 70

    Passionflower Tea 71

Desserts That Don't Disrupt Sleep 72

    Greek Yogurt with Honey and Almonds 72

    Dark Chocolate and Walnut Bites 73

    Banana Oat Cookies 74

    Chia Pudding with Berries 75

    Warm Baked Apples with Cinnamon 76

    Peanut Butter Banana Bites 77

    Coconut Date Rolls 78

    Pumpkin Pie Overnight Oats 79

    Avocado Chocolate Mousse 80

    Herbal Tea Gelatin Cups 81

Bonus: 28 Days Meal Plan 82

    Day 1 to Day 7 82

    Day 8 to Day 14 84

    Day 15 to Day 21 86

    Day 22 to Day 28 88

Conclusion 90

Special Bonus: A Gift of Flavor, Health, and Vitality 91

    Your Exclusive Bonuses Include: 91

    4 Additional Recipe Books: 91

    How to Access Your Bonus eBooks: 92

    First Book 93

    Second Book 94

    Third Book 95

Fourth Book..96

Introduction

Sleep is not a luxury. It is a fundamental pillar of health, as crucial as food, water, and air. Yet, in our fast-paced, always-on world, it's often the first thing we sacrifice. What if the secret to deep, restorative sleep wasn't just in bedtime routines or sleep hygiene—but on your plate? Imagine drifting into a peaceful slumber, waking up refreshed, all by making simple, delicious changes to your diet. This is the promise of the Why We Sleep Cookbook—where science meets nourishment for your best night's sleep.
Sleep is a biological necessity that governs how we think, feel, and function. Without enough quality rest, our bodies weaken, our minds fog, and our emotions fray. Chronic sleep deprivation has been linked to heart disease, diabetes, depression, and cognitive decline. But here's the good news: you can reclaim your nights—and your health—by harnessing the natural power of sleep-friendly foods.
In these pages, you will discover how nutrition profoundly influences your sleep cycle. The foods we eat can either disrupt or deepen our rest. Certain nutrients, such as magnesium, tryptophan, melatonin, and B vitamins, play a critical role in calming the nervous system, balancing hormones, and regulating the sleep-wake cycle. This cookbook is designed to provide you with recipes rich in these essential nutrients—delicious meals and snacks crafted to help you fall asleep faster, stay asleep longer, and wake up feeling rejuvenated.
But this isn't just a cookbook; it's a lifestyle guide. You'll learn how meal timing affects circadian rhythms, how caffeine and sugar sabotage sleep, and how light dinners rich in complex carbohydrates and lean proteins can pave the way for restful nights. Every recipe here is a step toward a more energized, focused, and vibrant you.
This book is for anyone who struggles to sleep, wakes up feeling groggy, or simply wants to optimize their health. It's for busy professionals, parents, students, and seniors—anyone ready to embrace the life-changing benefits of great sleep. And it all begins with what you eat.
So, let's begin this journey. Let's nourish the body in ways that heal, restore, and relax. Because better sleep starts in the kitchen—and so does a better life.

Welcome to the Why We Sleep Cookbook—your guide to delicious food and peaceful nights.

The Connection Between Sleep and Nutrition

Sleep and nutrition share a dynamic, interdependent relationship. Just as sleep influences how our bodies process and utilize food, the nutrients we consume can significantly affect our sleep patterns. Eating habits impact the production of hormones and neurotransmitters that regulate the sleep-wake cycle, such as melatonin and serotonin.

For instance, diets high in sugar and refined carbohydrates can disrupt sleep by causing fluctuations in blood sugar levels, leading to nighttime awakenings. Conversely, diets rich in fiber, lean proteins, healthy fats, and essential vitamins and minerals support deep, restorative sleep. The timing of meals also matters; eating heavy meals close to bedtime can impair digestion and lead to discomfort that disrupts sleep.

Nutrition doesn't just influence how we sleep; it shapes the quality and structure of our sleep cycles. By prioritizing sleep-friendly foods, you can enhance both the quantity and quality of your rest.

How Food Impacts Sleep Quality

The relationship between food and sleep quality is multifaceted, with factors like meal composition, timing, and portion size all playing roles. Here are some key ways in which food impacts sleep:

Regulation of Sleep Hormones
Certain foods support the body's production of melatonin and serotonin. Melatonin helps regulate circadian rhythms, signaling to the body when it's time to sleep, while serotonin plays a role in mood and sleep cycle regulation. Tryptophan-rich foods like turkey, nuts, and seeds promote serotonin synthesis, indirectly boosting melatonin production.

Blood Sugar Stability
Fluctuations in blood sugar levels can disrupt sleep. High-glycemic foods consumed late in the day can cause spikes in blood sugar, followed by rapid drops, which may lead to nighttime awakenings. Balanced meals with complex

carbohydrates, fiber, and healthy fats help maintain stable blood sugar levels, supporting uninterrupted sleep.

Magnesium and Relaxation
Magnesium plays a crucial role in activating the parasympathetic nervous system, responsible for promoting calm and relaxation. Foods rich in magnesium, such as dark leafy greens, bananas, and almonds, help relax muscles and prepare the body for restful sleep.

Meal Timing and Circadian Rhythms
Eating too close to bedtime can interfere with the body's circadian rhythms. Late-night meals may delay melatonin production, making it harder to fall asleep. Aim to have your last meal at least two to three hours before bedtime to align your digestive and sleep cycles.

Hydration
Dehydration can cause leg cramps and dry mouth, disrupting sleep. However, drinking excessive fluids before bed may increase nighttime bathroom trips. Balance is key—stay hydrated throughout the day and limit fluids an hour before bedtime.

The Science of Sleep-Friendly Nutrients

Certain nutrients are especially beneficial for promoting quality sleep. Incorporating these nutrients into your diet can make a significant difference in how well you rest:

Tryptophan
An essential amino acid, tryptophan is a precursor to serotonin and melatonin. Foods like turkey, eggs, cheese, and nuts are excellent sources.

Magnesium
Known for its calming properties, magnesium helps regulate neurotransmitters that prepare the body for sleep. Sources include spinach, pumpkin seeds, avocados, and dark chocolate.

Calcium
Calcium aids in the brain's use of tryptophan to manufacture melatonin. Dairy products, kale, and broccoli are rich in calcium.

Vitamin B6
Vitamin B6 assists in converting tryptophan to serotonin and melatonin. Bananas, chickpeas, and salmon are good sources.

Melatonin
Some foods contain natural melatonin, such as tart cherries, grapes, and tomatoes. Including these in your evening meal can help regulate your sleep-wake cycle.

Omega-3 Fatty Acids
Omega-3s, found in fatty fish like salmon and mackerel, support serotonin production, which promotes better sleep quality.

Creating an Evening Ritual with Food

An evening ritual centered around nourishing food can signal to your body that it's time to wind down. Here's how to design a routine that supports restful sleep:

Plan Light, Balanced Dinners
Choose meals that combine lean proteins, complex carbohydrates, and sleep-supportive nutrients. Avoid heavy, spicy, or high-fat meals that can cause digestive discomfort.

Example Recipe: Grilled salmon with quinoa and steamed spinach—a meal rich in omega-3s, magnesium, and tryptophan.

Incorporate Sleep-Inducing Snacks
If you feel hungry before bed, opt for light snacks that promote sleep, such as:
Greek yogurt with tart cherries (melatonin and tryptophan)
A banana with almond butter (magnesium and tryptophan)

Enjoy Herbal Teas
Calming herbal teas like chamomile, lavender, and valerian root can soothe the mind and body. Chamomile, for instance, contains apigenin, an antioxidant that binds to receptors in the brain to promote sleepiness.

Mindful Eating Practices
Slow down during your evening meal. Mindful eating reduces stress, enhances digestion, and prepares the body for rest. Focus on your food's flavors, textures, and aromas without distractions.

Set a Consistent Meal Schedule
Eat dinner at the same time each evening to support your circadian rhythm. Consistency signals to your body when to start winding down, making it easier to fall asleep.

The connection between sleep and nutrition is undeniable. By understanding how food influences sleep quality, incorporating sleep-friendly nutrients, and creating an intentional evening ritual with food, you can transform your nights—and your health. Each recipe and strategy in this cookbook is designed to guide you toward better rest through nourishment, ensuring you wake up each day feeling refreshed, energized, and ready to thrive.

Meal Planning for Sleep Optimization

Optimizing sleep starts well before bedtime. The food choices you make throughout the day, particularly in the evening, play a crucial role in supporting restful sleep. Thoughtful meal planning not only improves sleep quality but also supports overall health. This chapter explores how to structure meals for better sleep, offers weekly meal plans, and highlights foods to avoid for restful nights.

Meal Planning for Sleep Optimization

Effective meal planning for sleep focuses on incorporating foods rich in sleep-promoting nutrients while avoiding those that disrupt rest. Here's how to optimize your meal plan for better sleep:

Focus on Sleep-Supportive Nutrients

Include foods rich in tryptophan, magnesium, calcium, and B vitamins, which support the production of serotonin and melatonin. Lean proteins, whole grains, leafy greens, dairy, and nuts should be staples in your meal plan.

Balance Macronutrients

Balanced meals containing complex carbohydrates, healthy fats, and lean proteins promote stable blood sugar levels, preventing nighttime disruptions. Complex carbs help transport tryptophan to the brain, enhancing serotonin and melatonin production.

Timing Matters

Plan meals to align with your circadian rhythm. Eat heavier meals earlier in the day and opt for lighter dinners two to three hours before bedtime. Late-night eating can disrupt digestion and melatonin production.

Incorporate Relaxing Beverages

Warm, non-caffeinated drinks like chamomile tea or warm milk can become part of your evening ritual, signaling to the body that it's time to unwind.

Weekly Sleep-Friendly Meal Plans

Here's a sample week of meals designed to promote restful sleep

Monday
Breakfast: Oatmeal with almonds, chia seeds, and banana (rich in magnesium and tryptophan).
Lunch: Grilled chicken with quinoa and steamed broccoli.
Dinner: Baked salmon with sweet potato and sautéed spinach.
Evening Snack: Greek yogurt with tart cherries.

Tuesday
Breakfast: Blend spinach, banana, flaxseeds, and almond milk until smooth. Serve immediately and enjoy!
Lunch: Turkey wrap with whole-grain tortilla, lettuce, and avocado.
Dinner: Stir-fry tofu with brown rice and mixed vegetables.
Evening Snack: Herbal tea with a handful of walnuts.

Wednesday
Breakfast: Whole-grain toast with peanut butter and sliced bananas.
Lunch: Serve warm lentil soup with a slice of whole-grain bread on the side for a hearty and nutritious meal.
Dinner: Grilled trout with quinoa and asparagus.
Evening Snack: Cottage cheese with pineapple.

Thursday
Breakfast: Yogurt parfait with granola and berries.
Lunch: Chickpea salad with mixed greens, cherry tomatoes, and olive oil.
Dinner: Chicken and vegetable curry with brown rice.
Evening Snack: Warm chamomile tea.

Friday
Breakfast: Scrambled eggs with spinach and whole-grain toast.
Lunch: Tuna salad wrap with whole-grain tortilla.
Dinner: Baked cod with roasted vegetables and couscous.
Evening Snack: Banana with almond butter.

Saturday
Breakfast: Smoothie bowl with mixed berries and pumpkin seeds.
Lunch: Quinoa bowl with black beans, avocado, and grilled veggies.
Dinner: Serve grilled shrimp over a bed of zucchini noodles, topped with fresh pesto sauce for a light and flavorful dish.
Evening Snack: Herbal tea with dark chocolate (70% cocoa).

Sunday
Breakfast: Pancakes made with whole-grain flour, topped with fresh fruit.
Lunch: Turkey and avocado sandwich on whole-grain bread.
Dinner: Vegetable stir-fry with tofu and soba noodles.
Evening Snack: Warm milk with a dash of honey.

Tips for Structuring Evening Meals

Keep It Light and Balanced
Heavy meals can disrupt sleep by causing indigestion. Evening meals should be lighter than lunch, with a balance of complex carbs and lean proteins.

Incorporate Sleep-Promoting Ingredients
Include foods rich in magnesium (spinach, pumpkin seeds), tryptophan (turkey, nuts), and calcium (dairy, kale) to support melatonin production.

Mindful Meal Timing
Try to complete your dinner at least two to three hours before going to bed to support better digestion and sleep quality. This allows for proper digestion and aligns with the body's natural circadian rhythm.

Limit Sugary Desserts
Sugar can cause blood sugar spikes that interfere with sleep. If you crave something sweet, opt for fruit or dark chocolate.

Relaxation Rituals
Pair your evening meal with calming activities like reading or gentle stretching to signal to your body that it's time to wind down.

Foods to Avoid Before Bed

Certain foods and beverages can disrupt sleep. Here are key items to avoid:

Caffeine
Found in coffee, tea, chocolate, and some sodas, caffeine is a stimulant that can interfere with falling and staying asleep. Steer clear of caffeine for at least six hours before bedtime to promote restful sleep.

Alcohol
While alcohol might initially make you feel sleepy, it disrupts the later stages of the sleep cycle, leading to fragmented rest. Limit alcohol consumption, especially in the evening.

Heavy Spices
Spicy foods can cause heartburn and indigestion, disrupting sleep. Avoid heavily spiced meals before bed.

High-Fat Foods
Fatty foods take longer to digest, which can interfere with sleep quality. Opt for lighter meals with healthy fats like avocados and nuts.

Sugary Foods
High-sugar foods can cause blood sugar spikes and crashes, leading to restless nights. Choose naturally sweet options like fruit when craving a bedtime snack.

Large Meals
Large portions can cause discomfort and indigestion, making it harder to fall asleep. Keep dinners portion-controlled and balanced.

Meal planning is a powerful tool for sleep optimization. By understanding the impact of specific foods and nutrients, structuring evening meals mindfully, and avoiding sleep-disrupting items, you can transform your nights. The weekly meal plans and tips provided in this chapter are designed to support your body's natural rhythms, helping you fall asleep faster and wake up refreshed. Embrace these strategies and nourish your way to better sleep.

Lifestyle Practices for Better Sleep

Quality sleep is essential for overall well-being. While nutrition plays a crucial role in supporting restful sleep, lifestyle practices significantly influence sleep patterns as well. This chapter delves into combining nutrition with sleep hygiene practices, effective meditation and relaxation techniques, and ideal meal timing for optimal rest.

Lifestyle Practices for Better Sleep
To achieve restorative sleep, adopting healthy lifestyle habits is vital. These practices, when integrated with mindful nutrition, create a conducive environment for restful nights.

Establish a Consistent Sleep Schedule
Maintain a consistent sleep schedule by going to bed and waking up at the same time every day, including weekends. This helps regulate your circadian rhythm, making it easier to fall asleep and wake up naturally.

Create a Sleep-Inducing Environment
Ensure your bedroom is dark, quiet, and cool. Use blackout curtains, earplugs, or white noise machines as needed. A comfortable mattress and pillows tailored to your sleep style are also essential.

Limit Exposure to Screens Before Bed
Blue light from phones, tablets, and computers can suppress melatonin production, disrupting sleep. To promote better rest, turn off electronic devices at least an hour before bedtime.

Engage in Regular Physical Activity
Exercise promotes better sleep by reducing stress and tiring the body. Aim for at least 30 minutes of moderate activity daily, but avoid vigorous workouts close to bedtime.

Practice Evening Relaxation Techniques
Relaxing activities like reading, taking a warm bath, or listening to calming music can signal your body that it's time to wind down.

Combining Nutrition with Sleep Hygiene Practices

Nutrition and sleep hygiene go hand in hand. The timing, composition, and portion sizes of meals can complement good sleep hygiene practices.

Plan Balanced Evening Meals
Include foods rich in tryptophan, magnesium, and calcium, such as turkey, spinach, and dairy products. These nutrients support melatonin production and relaxation.

Stay Hydrated but Mindful
Drink enough water throughout the day but reduce fluid intake in the evening to minimize nighttime bathroom trips.

Limit Caffeine and Alcohol
Avoid caffeine after mid-afternoon and limit alcohol consumption in the evening. Both can disrupt the sleep cycle.

Mindful Evening Rituals
Pair your last meal with calming activities like journaling or gentle yoga to prepare your body and mind for rest.

Meditation and Relaxation Techniques After Dinner

Post-dinner relaxation techniques help calm the mind and body, facilitating better sleep.

Mindful Meditation
Spend 10-15 minutes in mindful meditation, focusing on your breath and letting go of the day's stress. This practice reduces anxiety and prepares the mind for restful sleep.

Progressive Muscle Relaxation (PMR)
PMR involves tensing and relaxing muscle groups, promoting physical relaxation. Start from your toes and work your way up, focusing on releasing tension.

Deep Breathing Exercises
Practice deep breathing techniques like the 4-7-8 method—inhale for 4 seconds, hold for 7 seconds, and exhale for 8 seconds. This technique calms the nervous system and promotes sleep.

Guided Imagery
Visualize peaceful scenes such as a beach or forest while listening to calming audio guides. Guided imagery shifts focus from stress to relaxation, easing the transition to sleep.

Aromatherapy
Use essential oils like lavender and chamomile, known for their sleep-inducing properties. Incorporate them into your evening routine through diffusers or pillow sprays.

Ideal Meal Timing for Optimal Sleep

The timing of your meals is just as crucial as the food choices you make. Proper meal timing supports your body's natural circadian rhythm and aids in better sleep quality.

Eat Dinner 2-3 Hours Before Bed
This allows time for digestion, reducing the risk of acid reflux and discomfort. Lighter dinners prevent the body from working hard to digest food during sleep.

Avoid Late-Night Snacks
While light snacks like bananas or yogurt can support sleep, avoid heavy, spicy, or sugary foods before bed, which can disrupt digestion and sleep.

Distribute Meals Evenly Throughout the Day
Balanced meals throughout the day maintain stable blood sugar levels, preventing nighttime hypoglycemia that can disrupt sleep.

Incorporate Small, Sleep-Promoting Snacks
If you're hungry before bed, opt for snacks like a small bowl of oatmeal, a handful of nuts, or herbal tea with honey. These foods promote relaxation without causing digestive issues.

Consistency in Meal Timing
Eat meals at consistent times each day. Regular meal schedules reinforce the circadian rhythm, supporting both digestion and sleep quality.

Achieving optimal sleep requires a holistic approach that combines mindful nutrition, effective sleep hygiene practices, and relaxation techniques. By adopting a consistent sleep schedule, creating a calming bedtime routine, incorporating sleep-supportive nutrients, and following ideal meal timing strategies, you can enhance sleep quality significantly. Embrace these comprehensive lifestyle practices and nourish your body and mind for restorative rest and overall well-being.

Morning Meals for Balanced Sleep

Banana and Almond Butter Oatmeal

Ingredients
Rolled oats: 1/2 cup (40g)
Banana (sliced): 1 medium (118g)
Almond butter: 1 tbsp (16g)
Chia seeds: 1 tsp (5g)
Low-fat milk: 1 cup (240ml)
Cinnamon: 1/4 tsp (0.5g)

Instructions
In a pot, bring the milk to a boil.
Add the oats and reduce to a simmer for 5 minutes, stirring occasionally.
Stir in cinnamon and chia seeds.
Top with banana slices and almond butter.

Nutritional Value
Calories: 350 kcal
Protein: 9g
Carbs: 50g
Fat: 12g
Fiber: 7g

Greek Yogurt with Berries and Walnuts

Ingredients
Greek yogurt (plain, 2%): 1 cup (245g)
Mixed berries: 1/2 cup (75g)
Walnuts (chopped): 1 oz (28g)
Honey: 1 tsp (7g)

Instructions
Combine yogurt, berries, and walnuts in a bowl.
Drizzle with honey before serving.

Nutritional Value
Calories: 320 kcal
Protein: 18g
Carbs: 22g
Fat: 16g
Fiber: 3g

Spinach and Feta Omelette

Ingredients
Eggs: 2 large (100g)
Spinach (fresh): 1 cup (30g)
Feta cheese (crumbled): 1 oz (28g)
Olive oil: 1 tsp (5ml)
Black pepper: to taste

Instructions
Warm olive oil in a skillet over medium heat.
Sauté spinach for 1-2 minutes.
Beat eggs with pepper and pour over spinach.
Sprinkle feta on top and cook until set.

Nutritional Value
Calories: 250 kcal
Protein: 18g
Carbs: 3g
Fat: 18g
Fiber: 1g

Avocado Toast with Whole Grain Bread

Ingredients
Whole grain bread: 1 slice (40g)
Avocado: 1/2 medium (68g)
Lemon juice: 1 tsp (5ml)
Salt and pepper: to taste

Instructions
Toast the bread.
Mash avocado with lemon juice, salt, and pepper.
Spread on toast and serve.

Nutritional Value
Calories: 270 kcal
Protein: 6g
Carbs: 28g
Fat: 15g
Fiber: 7g

Smoothie with Cherries, Spinach, and Almond Milk

Ingredients
Frozen cherries: 1/2 cup (70g)
Spinach (fresh): 1 cup (30g)
Almond milk (unsweetened): 1 cup (240ml)
Chia seeds: 1 tbsp (12g)

Instructions
Blend all ingredients until smooth.
Serve immediately.

Nutritional Value
Calories: 200 kcal
Protein: 4g
Carbs: 25g
Fat: 9g
Fiber: 6g

Quinoa Breakfast Bowl with Nuts and Fruits

Ingredients
Cooked quinoa: 1/2 cup (93g)
Almonds (sliced): 1 oz (28g)
Blueberries: 1/2 cup (74g)
Low-fat Greek yogurt: 1/2 cup (122g)

Instructions
Layer quinoa, yogurt, berries, and almonds in a bowl.
Serve chilled or at room temperature.

Nutritional Value
Calories: 330 kcal
Protein: 15g
Carbs: 30g
Fat: 15g
Fiber: 5g

Whole Wheat Pancakes with Banana and Honey

Ingredients
Whole wheat flour: 1/2 cup (60g)
Baking powder: 1 tsp (4g)
Egg: 1 large (50g)
Banana (sliced): 1 medium (118g)
Honey: 1 tsp (7g)
Low-fat milk: 1/2 cup (120ml)

Instructions
Mix flour and baking powder.
Add egg and milk to form batter.
Cook pancakes on a skillet and top with banana and honey.

Nutritional Value
Calories: 320 kcal
Protein: 10g
Carbs: 45g
Fat: 9g
Fiber: 5g

Cottage Cheese and Pineapple Bowl

Ingredients
Low-fat cottage cheese: 1 cup (210g)
Pineapple chunks: 1/2 cup (82g)
Ground flaxseeds: 1 tbsp (7g)

Instructions
Combine cottage cheese, pineapple, and flaxseeds in a bowl. Serve immediately.

Nutritional Value
Calories: 250 kcal
Protein: 20g
Carbs: 18g
Fat: 9g
Fiber: 3g

Scrambled Eggs with Smoked Salmon and Arugula

Ingredients
Eggs: 2 large (100g)
Smoked salmon: 2 oz (56g)
Arugula: 1 cup (20g)
Olive oil: 1 tsp (5ml)

Instructions
Beat eggs and scramble in olive oil over medium heat.
Top with smoked salmon and arugula.

Nutritional Value
Calories: 300 kcal
Protein: 22g
Carbs: 2g
Fat: 22g
Fiber: 1g

Tofu and Veggie Breakfast Wrap

Ingredients
Firm tofu (crumbled): 1/2 cup (126g)
Whole wheat tortilla: 1 medium (50g)
Bell pepper (diced): 1/2 cup (75g)
Spinach (fresh): 1/2 cup (15g)
Olive oil: 1 tsp (5ml)

Instructions
Sauté tofu and vegetables in olive oil for 5 minutes. Wrap in tortilla and serve warm.

Nutritional Value
Calories: 320 kcal
Protein: 18g
Carbs: 25g
Fat: 14g
Fiber: 5g

Energizing Lunches Without Disrupting Sleep

Grilled Chicken and Quinoa Salad

Ingredients
Grilled chicken breast: 4 oz (113g)
Cooked quinoa: 1 cup (185g)
Cherry tomatoes (halved): 1/2 cup (75g)
Cucumber (diced): 1/2 cup (52g)
Olive oil: 1 tbsp (15ml)
Lemon juice: 1 tbsp (15ml)
Fresh parsley (chopped): 1 tbsp (4g)

Instructions
Combine quinoa, tomatoes, cucumber, and parsley in a bowl.
Top with grilled chicken slices.
Drizzle olive oil and lemon juice before serving.

Nutritional Value
Calories: 450 kcal
Protein: 32g
Carbs: 35g
Fat: 18g
Fiber: 5g

Lentil and Vegetable Stew

Ingredients
Cooked lentils: 1 cup (198g)
Carrot (sliced): 1/2 cup (61g)
Celery (chopped): 1/2 cup (50g)
Spinach (fresh): 1 cup (30g)
Olive oil: 1 tsp (5ml)
Vegetable broth: 2 cups (480ml)

Instructions
Sauté carrots and celery in olive oil for 3 minutes.
Add lentils and broth, simmer for 10 minutes.
Stir in spinach and cook for 2 minutes before serving.

Nutritional Value
Calories: 320 kcal
Protein: 18g
Carbs: 45g
Fat: 5g
Fiber: 12g

Turkey and Avocado Wrap

Ingredients
Whole wheat tortilla: 1 medium (50g)
Sliced turkey breast: 3 oz (85g)
Avocado (sliced): 1/2 medium (68g)
Baby spinach: 1/2 cup (15g)
Greek yogurt (plain): 1 tbsp (15g)

Instructions
Spread yogurt on the tortilla.
Add turkey, avocado, and spinach.
Roll tightly and slice in half before serving.

Nutritional Value
Calories: 350 kcal
Protein: 25g
Carbs: 28g
Fat: 15g
Fiber: 6g

Chickpea and Spinach Stir-Fry

Ingredients
Cooked chickpeas: 1 cup (164g)
Spinach (fresh): 2 cups (60g)
Garlic (minced): 1 clove (3g)
Olive oil: 1 tsp (5ml)
Lemon juice: 1 tbsp (15ml)

Instructions
Warm olive oil in a pan and sauté garlic for 1 minute until fragrant.
Add chickpeas and stir-fry for 3 minutes.
Stir in spinach and lemon juice; cook until wilted.

Nutritional Value
Calories: 320 kcal
Protein: 12g
Carbs: 40g
Fat: 10g
Fiber: 10g

Salmon and Brown Rice Bowl

Ingredients
Grilled salmon: 4 oz (113g)
Brown rice (cooked): 1 cup (195g)
Steamed broccoli: 1 cup (156g)
Soy sauce (low sodium): 1 tbsp (15ml)

Instructions
Place brown rice in a bowl.
Top with grilled salmon and steamed broccoli.
Drizzle soy sauce before serving.

Nutritional Value
Calories: 480 kcal
Protein: 28g
Carbs: 40g
Fat: 18g
Fiber: 5g

Hummus and Vegetable Pita

Ingredients
Whole wheat pita: 1 medium (60g)
Hummus: 1/4 cup (60g)
Bell peppers (sliced): 1/2 cup (75g)
Cucumber (sliced): 1/2 cup (52g)
Red onion (sliced): 1/4 cup (28g)

Instructions
Spread hummus inside the pita.
Stuff with vegetables and serve immediately.

Nutritional Value
Calories: 350 kcal
Protein: 12g
Carbs: 40g
Fat: 12g
Fiber: 8g

Grilled Veggie and Goat Cheese Sandwich

Ingredients
Whole grain bread: 2 slices (80g)
Zucchini (grilled): 1/2 cup (57g)
Eggplant (grilled): 1/2 cup (50g)
Goat cheese: 1 oz (28g)
Olive oil: 1 tsp (5ml)

Instructions
Spread goat cheese on bread slices.
Add grilled vegetables and press into a sandwich.
Grill until golden brown.

Nutritional Value
Calories: 400 kcal
Protein: 14g
Carbs: 42g
Fat: 18g
Fiber: 6g

Shrimp and Avocado Salad

Ingredients
Cooked shrimp: 4 oz (113g)
Avocado (sliced): 1/2 medium (68g)
Mixed greens: 2 cups (85g)
Olive oil: 1 tbsp (15ml)
Lime juice: 1 tbsp (15ml)

Instructions
Arrange mixed greens, shrimp, and avocado in a bowl.
Drizzle with olive oil and lime juice.

Nutritional Value
Calories: 370 kcal
Protein: 25g
Carbs: 12g
Fat: 22g
Fiber: 7g

Sweet Potato and Black Bean Bowl

Ingredients
Roasted sweet potato: 1 cup (133g)
Black beans (cooked): 1/2 cup (120g)
Avocado (sliced): 1/2 medium (68g)
Lime juice: 1 tbsp (15ml)

Instructions
Combine sweet potato, black beans, and avocado in a bowl. Drizzle with lime juice before serving.

Nutritional Value
Calories: 400 kcal
Protein: 12g
Carbs: 48g
Fat: 14g
Fiber: 10g

Chicken and Vegetable Stir-Fry

Ingredients
Chicken breast (sliced): 4 oz (113g)
Bell peppers (sliced): 1 cup (150g)
Broccoli (florets): 1 cup (91g)
Olive oil: 1 tbsp (15ml)
Soy sauce (low sodium): 1 tbsp (15ml)

Instructions
Heat olive oil in a skillet.
Sauté chicken until cooked through.
Add vegetables and cook until tender.
Drizzle soy sauce and serve

Nutritional Value
Calories: 420 kcal
Protein: 30g
Carbs: 20g
Fat: 18g
Fiber: 5g

Sleep-Promoting Dinners

Grilled Salmon with Quinoa and Asparagus

Ingredients
Salmon fillet: 6 oz
Quinoa: 1 cup (cooked)
Asparagus: 1 cup
Olive oil: 1 tbsp
Lemon juice: 1 tbsp
Salt and pepper: to taste

Instructions
Preheat the grill to medium heat.
Place the salmon on a baking sheet and season with salt, pepper, and a squeeze of lemon juice.
Grill salmon for 5–6 minutes on each side.
Steam asparagus for 4–5 minutes.
Drizzle with olive oil and garnish with fresh parsley and lemon wedges before serving.

Nutritional Value
Calories: 480 kcal
Protein: 35g
Carbs: 25g
Fat: 25g

Turkey and Sweet Potato Bowl

Ingredients
Ground turkey: 6 oz
Sweet potato: 1 cup (cubed)
Olive oil: 1 tbsp
Spinach: 1 cup
Garlic: 1 clove (minced)

Instructions
Sauté garlic in olive oil for 1 minute.
Add ground turkey and cook until browned.
Roast sweet potatoes at 400°F for 20 minutes.
Combine turkey, sweet potatoes, and spinach in a bowl.

Nutritional Value
Calories: 500 kcal
Protein: 38g
Carbs: 30g
Fat: 20g

Tofu and Vegetable Stir-Fry

Ingredients
Firm tofu: 6 oz
Broccoli: 1 cup
Bell peppers: 1 cup (sliced)
Soy sauce: 2 tbsp
Sesame oil: 1 tbsp

Instructions
Sauté tofu in sesame oil until golden.
Add vegetables and stir-fry for 5 minutes.
Stir well to combine and serve immediately with steamed rice or noodles.

Nutritional Value
Calories: 420 kcal
Protein: 25g
Carbs: 20g
Fat: 22g

Chicken and Brown Rice with Kale

Ingredients
Chicken breast: 6 oz
Brown rice: 1 cup (cooked)
Kale: 1 cup
Olive oil: 1 tbsp
Lemon juice: 1 tbsp

Instructions
Grill chicken until cooked through.
Sauté kale in olive oil for 3–4 minutes.
Serve chicken on brown rice with kale on the side.

Nutritional Value
Calories: 480 kcal
Protein: 40g
Carbs: 28g
Fat: 18g

Lentil and Vegetable Stew

Ingredients
Lentils: 1 cup (cooked)
Carrots: 1 cup (chopped)
Celery: 1 cup (chopped)
Vegetable broth: 2 cups
Olive oil: 1 tbsp

Instructions
Sauté vegetables in olive oil for 5 minutes.
Add lentils and broth; simmer for 20 minutes.

Nutritional Value
Calories: 390 kcal
Protein: 22g
Carbs: 35g
Fat: 12g

Shrimp and Avocado Salad

Ingredients
Shrimp: 6 oz (cooked)
Avocado: 1/2 (sliced)
Mixed greens: 2 cups
Olive oil: 1 tbsp
Lime juice: 1 tbsp

Instructions
Toss shrimp, avocado, and greens in olive oil and lime juice.

Nutritional Value
Calories: 420 kcal
Protein: 30g
Carbs: 15g
Fat: 22g

Cod with Lemon and Steamed Veggies

Ingredients
Cod fillet: 6 oz
Zucchini: 1 cup (sliced)
Carrots: 1 cup (sliced)
Lemon: 1/2 (sliced)

Instructions
Bake cod at 375°F for 15 minutes with lemon slices.
Steam vegetables for 5 minutes.

Nutritional Value
Calories: 350 kcal
Protein: 32g
Carbs: 20g
Fat: 10g

Chickpea and Spinach Curry

Ingredients
Chickpeas: 1 cup (cooked)
Spinach: 2 cups
Coconut milk: 1 cup
Curry powder: 1 tbsp

Instructions
Sauté chickpeas and curry powder for 2 minutes.
Add spinach and coconut milk; simmer for 10 minutes.

Nutritional Value
Calories: 450 kcal
Protein: 20g
Carbs: 35g
Fat: 22g

Baked Chicken with Sweet Potato and Green Beans

Ingredients
Chicken thigh: 6 oz
Sweet potato: 1 cup (cubed)
Green beans: 1 cup
Olive oil: 1 tbsp

Instructions
Bake chicken at 375°F for 25 minutes.
Roast sweet potatoes for 20 minutes.
Steam green beans for 5 minutes.

Nutritional Value
Calories: 500 kcal
Protein: 35g
Carbs: 30g
Fat: 22g

Quinoa-Stuffed Bell Peppers

Ingredients
Bell peppers: 2 (halved and seeded)
Quinoa: 1 cup (cooked)
Black beans: 1/2 cup
Corn: 1/2 cup
Cheddar cheese: 1/4 cup (shredded)

Instructions
Mix quinoa, black beans, and corn.
Stuff mixture into bell peppers; top with cheese.
Bake at 375°F for 20 minutes.

Nutritional Value
Calories: 480 kcal
Protein: 25g
Carbs: 35g
Fat: 20g

Soothing Snacks for a Restful Night

Banana and Almond Butter Bites

Ingredients
Banana: 1 medium (sliced)
Almond butter: 2 tbsp

Instructions
Spread almond butter on banana slices.
Stack slices to make small sandwiches.

Nutritional Value
Calories: 210 kcal
Protein: 4g
Carbs: 27g
Fat: 10g

Greek Yogurt with Honey and Walnuts

Ingredients
Greek yogurt (plain, 2%): 1 cup
Honey: 1 tbsp
Walnuts: 2 tbsp (chopped)

Instructions
Mix honey and walnuts into the yogurt.

Nutritional Value
Calories: 250 kcal
Protein: 15g
Carbs: 20g
Fat: 12g

Chamomile Tea with Whole-Grain Crackers and Cheese

Ingredients
Chamomile tea: 1 cup (brewed)
Whole-grain crackers: 5 pieces
Cheddar cheese: 1 oz (sliced)

Instructions
Brew chamomile tea.
Serve crackers with cheese on the side.

Nutritional Value
Calories: 220 kcal
Protein: 8g
Carbs: 18g
Fat: 12g

Kiwi and Pumpkin Seeds Bowl

Ingredients
Kiwi: 2 medium (sliced)
Pumpkin seeds: 2 tbsp

Instructions
Combine kiwi slices and pumpkin seeds in a bowl.

Nutritional Value
Calories: 180 kcal
Protein: 4g
Carbs: 24g
Fat: 7g

Warm Oatmeal with Cinnamon and Almonds

Ingredients
Oats: 1/2 cup (dry)
Almonds: 2 tbsp (sliced)
Cinnamon: 1/2 tsp
Milk (dairy or plant-based): 1 cup

Instructions
Cook oats with milk over medium heat.
Stir in cinnamon and top with almonds.

Nutritional Value
Calories: 260 kcal
Protein: 7g
Carbs: 30g
Fat: 12g

Apple Slices with Peanut Butter

Ingredients
Apple: 1 medium (sliced)
Peanut butter: 2 tbsp

Instructions
Spread peanut butter on apple slices.

Nutritional Value
Calories: 240 kcal
Protein: 4g
Carbs: 30g
Fat: 12g

Cottage Cheese with Pineapple

Ingredients
Cottage cheese (low-fat): 1 cup
Pineapple chunks: 1/2 cup

Instructions
Combine cottage cheese and pineapple in a bowl.

Nutritional Value
Calories: 220 kcal
Protein: 20g
Carbs: 18g
Fat: 6g

Avocado Toast on Whole-Grain Bread

Ingredients
Whole-grain bread: 1 slice
Avocado: 1/2 (mashed)
Lemon juice: 1 tsp
Salt: a pinch

Instructions
Toast the bread.
Spread avocado on toast and drizzle with lemon juice.

Nutritional Value
Calories: 220 kcal
Protein: 5g
Carbs: 20g
Fat: 14g

Herbal Tea with Dark Chocolate

Ingredients
Herbal tea (e.g., chamomile or valerian root): 1 cup (brewed)
Dark chocolate (70% cacao): 1 oz

Instructions
Brew herbal tea.
Serve with dark chocolate on the side.

Nutritional Value
Calories: 170 kcal
Protein: 2g
Carbs: 12g
Fat: 12g

Warm Milk with Nutmeg

Ingredients
Milk (dairy or plant-based): 1 cup
Nutmeg: a pinch

Instructions
Warm the milk without boiling.
Sprinkle nutmeg on top before serving.

Nutritional Value
Calories: 150 kcal
Protein: 8g
Carbs: 12g
Fat: 7g

Calming Teas and Smoothies

Chamomile Lavender Tea

Ingredients
Dried chamomile flowers: 1 tbsp
Dried lavender buds: 1 tsp
Water: 1 cup

Instructions
Boil water and pour over chamomile and lavender.
Steep for 5–7 minutes, strain, and serve.

Nutritional Value
Calories: 0 kcal
Protein: 0g
Carbs: 0g
Fat: 0g

Banana Almond Sleep Smoothie

Ingredients
Banana: 1 medium
Almond milk: 1 cup
Honey: 1 tsp
Ground cinnamon: 1/4 tsp

Instructions
Blend all ingredients until smooth.

Nutritional Value
Calories: 190 kcal
Protein: 3g
Carbs: 32g
Fat: 5g

Valerian Root Tea

Ingredients
Valerian root: 1 tsp (dried)
Water: 1 cup

Instructions
Boil water and pour over valerian root. Steep for 10 minutes, strain, and serve.

Nutritional Value
Calories: 0 kcal
Protein: 0g
Carbs: 0g
Fat: 0g

Kiwi and Spinach Sleep Smoothie

Ingredients
Kiwi: 2 medium (peeled)
Spinach: 1 cup
Greek yogurt: 1/2 cup
Water: 1/2 cup

Instructions
Blend all ingredients until smooth.

Nutritional Value
Calories: 160 kcal
Protein: 10g
Carbs: 24g
Fat: 2g

Peppermint Herbal Tea

Ingredients
Fresh peppermint leaves: 1 tbsp
Water: 1 cup

Instructions
Boil water and pour over peppermint leaves. Steep for 5 minutes, strain, and serve.

Nutritional Value
Calories: 0 kcal
Protein: 0g
Carbs: 0g
Fat: 0g

Tart Cherry and Almond Smoothie

Ingredients
Tart cherry juice: 1/2 cup
Almond milk: 1/2 cup
Greek yogurt: 1/4 cup

Instructions
Blend all ingredients until smooth.

Nutritional Value
Calories: 150 kcal
Protein: 6g
Carbs: 20g
Fat: 4g

Lemon Balm Tea

Ingredients
Lemon balm leaves: 1 tbsp (fresh or dried)
Water: 1 cup

Instructions
Boil water and pour over lemon balm leaves.
Steep for 5–7 minutes, strain, and serve.

Nutritional Value
Calories: 0 kcal
Protein: 0g
Carbs: 0g
Fat: 0g

Golden Milk Smoothie

Ingredients
Turmeric powder: 1/2 tsp
Cinnamon: 1/4 tsp
Ginger powder: 1/4 tsp
Honey: 1 tsp
Warm almond milk: 1 cup

Instructions
Blend all ingredients until smooth and serve warm.

Nutritional Value
Calories: 140 kcal
Protein: 2g
Carbs: 16g
Fat: 6g

Ashwagandha Sleep Smoothie

Ingredients
Banana: 1 medium
Almond milk: 1 cup
Ashwagandha powder: 1/4 tsp
Honey: 1 tsp

Instructions
Blend all ingredients until smooth.

Nutritional Value
Calories: 180 kcal
Protein: 3g
Carbs: 30g
Fat: 5g

Passionflower Tea

Ingredients
Dried passionflower: 1 tsp
Water: 1 cup

Instructions
Boil water and pour over passionflower. Steep for 10 minutes, strain, and serve.

Nutritional Value
Calories: 0 kcal
Protein: 0g
Carbs: 0g
Fat: 0g

Desserts That Don't Disrupt Sleep

Greek Yogurt with Honey and Almonds

Ingredients
Greek yogurt (unsweetened): 1 cup
Honey: 1 tsp
Sliced almonds: 1 tbsp

Instructions
Spoon the Greek yogurt into a bowl.
Drizzle with honey and top with almonds.

Nutritional Value
Calories: 180 kcal
Protein: 12g
Carbs: 16g
Fat: 6g

Dark Chocolate and Walnut Bites

Ingredients
Dark chocolate (70% cacao): 1 oz
Walnuts: 1 oz

Instructions
Melt dark chocolate and coat walnuts.
Refrigerate until chocolate hardens.

Nutritional Value
Calories: 200 kcal
Protein: 3g
Carbs: 10g
Fat: 16g

Banana Oat Cookies

Ingredients
Ripe bananas: 2 medium
Rolled oats: 1 cup
Cinnamon: 1/2 tsp

Instructions
Preheat oven to 350°F (175°C).
Mash bananas and mix with oats and cinnamon.
Scoop onto baking sheet and bake for 15 minutes.

Nutritional Value
Calories: 120 kcal (per cookie)
Protein: 2g
Carbs: 20g
Fat: 2g

Chia Pudding with Berries

Ingredients
Chia seeds: 3 tbsp
Almond milk: 1 cup
Mixed berries: 1/2 cup

Instructions
Mix chia seeds and almond milk.
Refrigerate overnight and top with berries before serving.

Nutritional Value
Calories: 250 kcal
Protein: 5g
Carbs: 20g
Fat: 12g

Warm Baked Apples with Cinnamon

Ingredients
Apples: 2 medium
Cinnamon: 1 tsp
Maple syrup: 1 tbsp

Instructions
Preheat oven to 375°F (190°C).
Core apples, drizzle with maple syrup, and sprinkle with cinnamon.
Bake for 20 minutes.

Nutritional Value
Calories: 150 kcal
Protein: 0g
Carbs: 36g
Fat: 0g

Peanut Butter Banana Bites

Ingredients
Banana: 1 medium
Peanut butter: 2 tbsp

Instructions
Slice banana and spread peanut butter between two slices.
Chill in the freezer for 10 minutes before serving.

Nutritional Value
Calories: 210 kcal
Protein: 5g
Carbs: 27g
Fat: 9g

Coconut Date Rolls

Ingredients
Medjool dates: 6
Shredded coconut (unsweetened): 2 tbsp

Instructions
Pit the dates and roll them in shredded coconut. Chill before serving.

Nutritional Value
Calories: 140 kcal (per roll)
Protein: 1g
Carbs: 36g
Fat: 2g

Pumpkin Pie Overnight Oats

Ingredients
Rolled oats: 1/2 cup
Pumpkin puree: 1/4 cup
Almond milk: 1/2 cup
Cinnamon: 1/4 tsp
Nutmeg: 1/8 tsp

Instructions
Mix all ingredients in a jar and chill in the refrigerator overnight.

Nutritional Value
Calories: 220 kcal
Protein: 5g
Carbs: 36g
Fat: 5g

Avocado Chocolate Mousse

Ingredients
Ripe avocado: 1 medium
Cocoa powder: 2 tbsp
Honey: 1 tbsp
Vanilla extract: 1/2 tsp

Instructions
Blend all ingredients until smooth.
Chill for 1 hour before serving.

Nutritional Value
Calories: 240 kcal
Protein: 3g
Carbs: 20g
Fat: 16g

Herbal Tea Gelatin Cups

Ingredients
Chamomile tea (brewed): 2 cups
Gelatin powder: 2 tbsp
Honey: 1 tbsp

Instructions
Dissolve gelatin in warm tea.
Add honey, pour into molds, and refrigerate until set.

Nutritional Value
Calories: 40 kcal (per cup)
Protein: 4g
Carbs: 5g
Fat: 0g

Bonus: 28 Days Meal Plan

Day 1 to Day 7

Day 1
Breakfast: Greek Yogurt with Honey and Almonds
Lunch: Quinoa Salad with Chickpeas and Avocado
Dinner: Baked Salmon with Steamed Broccoli
Snack: Chia Pudding with Berries
Tea/Smoothie: Chamomile Lavender Tea
Dessert: Warm Baked Apples with Cinnamon

Day 2
Breakfast: Overnight Oats with Almond Butter
Lunch: Turkey and Hummus Wrap
Dinner: Grilled Chicken with Sweet Potato Mash
Snack: Peanut Butter Banana Bites
Tea/Smoothie: Banana Almond Smoothie
Dessert: Banana Oat Cookies

Day 3
Breakfast: Avocado Toast with Poached Egg
Lunch: Lentil Soup with Whole Grain Bread
Dinner: Quinoa and Veggie Stir-Fry
Snack: Dark Chocolate and Walnut Bites
Tea/Smoothie: Valerian Root Tea
Dessert: Coconut Date Rolls

Day 4
Breakfast: Berry Smoothie Bowl
Lunch: Grilled Shrimp Salad with Lemon Dressing
Dinner: Baked Cod with Asparagus
Snack: Pumpkin Pie Overnight Oats
Tea/Smoothie: Herbal Tea Gelatin Cups
Dessert: Avocado Chocolate Mousse

Day 5
Breakfast: Greek Yogurt with Mixed Berries
Lunch: Chicken Caesar Salad (light dressing)
Dinner: Stuffed Bell Peppers
Snack: Apple Slices with Almond Butter
Tea/Smoothie: Warm Chamomile Tea
Dessert: Peanut Butter Banana Bites

Day 6
Breakfast: Scrambled Eggs with Spinach
Lunch: Tuna Salad Wrap
Dinner: Grilled Turkey Breast with Green Beans
Snack: Banana Oat Cookies
Tea/Smoothie: Peppermint Tea
Dessert: Chia Pudding with Berries

Day 7
Breakfast: Oatmeal with Walnuts and Cinnamon
Lunch: Vegetable Stir-Fry with Tofu
Dinner: Lemon Herb Chicken with Quinoa
Snack: Dark Chocolate and Walnut Bites
Tea/Smoothie: Banana Almond Smoothie
Dessert: Warm Baked Apples with Cinnamon

Day 8 to Day 14

Day 8
Breakfast: Berry Smoothie Bowl
Lunch: Mediterranean Chickpea Salad
Dinner: Baked Trout with Wild Rice
Snack: Peanut Butter Banana Bites
Tea/Smoothie: Lavender Chamomile Tea
Dessert: Coconut Date Rolls

Day 9
Breakfast: Greek Yogurt with Honey and Almonds
Lunch: Spinach and Feta Wrap
Dinner: Turkey Meatballs with Zucchini Noodles
Snack: Pumpkin Pie Overnight Oats
Tea/Smoothie: Herbal Tea Gelatin Cups
Dessert: Avocado Chocolate Mousse

Day 10
Breakfast: Scrambled Eggs with Tomatoes
Lunch: Chicken and Avocado Sandwich
Dinner: Roasted Veggie and Lentil Stew
Snack: Apple Slices with Almond Butter
Tea/Smoothie: Peppermint Tea
Dessert: Banana Oat Cookies

Day 11
Breakfast: Overnight Oats with Blueberries
Lunch: Quinoa and Kale Salad
Dinner: Grilled Salmon with Spinac
Snack: Chia Pudding with Berries
Tea/Smoothie: Valerian Root Tea
Dessert: Peanut Butter Banana Bites

Day 12
Breakfast: Avocado Toast with Poached Egg
Lunch: Sweet Potato and Black Bean Tacos
Dinner: Herb Chicken with Brown Rice
Snack: Dark Chocolate and Walnut Bites
Tea/Smoothie: Banana Almond Smoothie
Dessert: Warm Baked Apples with Cinnamon

Day 13
Breakfast: Oatmeal with Almond Butter
Lunch: Grilled Veggie Wrap
Dinner: Lemon Garlic Shrimp with Asparagus
Snack: Coconut Date Rolls
Tea/Smoothie: Herbal Tea Gelatin Cups
Dessert: Avocado Chocolate Mousse

Day 14
Breakfast: Greek Yogurt with Mixed Berries
Lunch: Tofu and Veggie Stir-Fry
Dinner: Roasted Chicken with Sweet Potatoes
Snack: Apple Slices with Almond Butter
Tea/Smoothie: Peppermint Tea
Dessert: Banana Oat Cookies

Day 15 to Day 21

Day 15
Breakfast: Greek Yogurt with Honey and Walnuts
Lunch: Chickpea and Spinach Wrap
Dinner: Grilled Tilapia with Brown Rice and Broccoli
Snack: Almond Butter Energy Balls
Tea/Smoothie: Lemon Balm Tea
Dessert: Baked Pears with Cinnamon

Day 16
Breakfast: Oatmeal with Pumpkin Seeds and Blueberries
Lunch: Turkey and Avocado Salad
Dinner: Quinoa Stuffed Bell Peppers
Snack: Greek Yogurt with Honey
Tea/Smoothie: Golden Milk Smoothie
Dessert: Dark Chocolate Dipped Strawberries

Day 17
Breakfast: Scrambled Eggs with Whole Grain Toast
Lunch: Roasted Veggie and Quinoa Bowl
Dinner: Baked Cod with Garlic Mashed Cauliflower
Snack: Apple Slices with Cashew Butter
Tea/Smoothie: Chamomile Tea
Dessert: Coconut Chia Pudding

Day 18
Breakfast: Overnight Oats with Almond Butter and Banana
Lunch: Lentil and Sweet Potato Stew
Dinner: Lemon Herb Grilled Chicken with Asparagus
Snack: Pumpkin Spice Protein Bites
Tea/Smoothie: Valerian Root Tea
Dessert: Baked Apples with Raisins

Day 19
Breakfast: Berry Smoothie with Spinach and Flaxseeds
Lunch: Tuna Salad Wrap with Avocado
Dinner: Roasted Turkey Breast with Green Beans
Snack: Hummus with Cucumber Slices
Tea/Smoothie: Peppermint Tea
Dessert: Dark Chocolate and Walnut Clusters

Day 20
Breakfast: Avocado Toast with Poached Egg
Lunch: Grilled Chicken and Kale Salad
Dinner: Shrimp and Vegetable Stir-Fry
Snack: Peanut Butter Banana Bites
Tea/Smoothie: Banana Almond Smoothie
Dessert: Baked Pears with Cinnamon

Day 21
Breakfast: Greek Yogurt with Mixed Berries and Chia Seeds
Lunch: Tofu and Vegetable Wrap
Dinner: Herb-Crusted Salmon with Steamed Spinach
Snack: Almond Butter Energy Balls
Tea/Smoothie: Chamomile Lavender Tea
Dessert: Coconut Chia Pudding

Day 22 to Day 28

Day 22
Breakfast: Oatmeal with Walnuts and Maple Syrup
Lunch: Grilled Chicken Caesar Wrap
Dinner: Baked Trout with Roasted Brussels Sprouts
Snack: Greek Yogurt with Honey and Almonds
Tea/Smoothie: Lemon Balm Tea
Dessert: Avocado Chocolate Mousse

Day 23
Breakfast: Smoothie Bowl with Berries and Flaxseeds
Lunch: Lentil and Kale Soup
Dinner: Baked Turkey Meatballs with Zucchini Noodles
Snack: Peanut Butter Banana Bites
Tea/Smoothie: Golden Milk Smoothie
Dessert: Dark Chocolate Dipped Strawberries

Day 24
Breakfast: Scrambled Eggs with Spinach and Tomatoes
Lunch: Quinoa and Veggie Stir-Fry
Dinner: Grilled Chicken with Wild Rice and Green Beans
Snack: Chia Pudding with Fresh Berries
Tea/Smoothie: Peppermint Tea
Dessert: Warm Baked Apples with Cinnamon

Day 25
Breakfast: Avocado Toast with Sliced Tomato
Lunch: Mediterranean Chickpea Salad
Dinner: Grilled Shrimp with Lemon Garlic Sauce
Snack: Dark Chocolate and Walnut Bites
Tea/Smoothie: Valerian Root Tea
Dessert: Coconut Date Rolls

Day 26
Breakfast: Almond Butter and Chia Seed Overnight Oats
Lunch: Grilled Veggie and Hummus Wrap
Dinner: Lemon Garlic Baked Cod with Broccoli
Snack: Apple Slices with Almond Butter
Tea/Smoothie: Chamomile Tea
Dessert: Avocado Chocolate Mousse

Day 27
Breakfast: Greek Yogurt with Pumpkin Seeds and Berries
Lunch: Sweet Potato and Black Bean Tacos
Dinner: Baked Chicken Thighs with Quinoa and Kale
Snack: Peanut Butter Banana Bites
Tea/Smoothie: Banana Almond Smoothie
Dessert: Baked Pears with Cinnamon

Day 28
Breakfast: Oatmeal with Cinnamon and Walnuts
Lunch: Grilled Salmon Salad with Lemon Vinaigrette
Dinner: Stuffed Bell Peppers with Quinoa and Turkey
Snack: Dark Chocolate and Walnut Clusters
Tea/Smoothie: Peppermint Tea
Dessert: Coconut Chia Pudding

Conclusion

As you reach the end of this transformative journey through the Why We Sleep Cookbook, it's clear that the connection between nutrition and restorative sleep is profound. The recipes, meal plans, and lifestyle tips provided throughout this book are more than just guidance—they represent a holistic approach to achieving deep, rejuvenating rest every night.

By integrating sleep-friendly nutrients, thoughtful meal timing, and relaxing evening rituals, you are not only enhancing the quality of your sleep but also enriching your overall health and well-being. Each carefully crafted recipe and meal plan was designed with one purpose in mind: to help you unlock the power of sleep through nourishing, delicious food choices.

Remember, quality sleep is not a luxury—it's a necessity. It is the foundation upon which mental clarity, physical vitality, and emotional resilience are built. As you continue to incorporate the strategies and meals from this book into your daily routine, you will experience better energy levels, improved focus, and a greater sense of balance in your life.

Let this book serve as your ongoing companion in your pursuit of optimal rest. Experiment with the recipes, adjust the meal plans to fit your needs, and embrace the calming practices that signal your body and mind that it's time to unwind. In doing so, you are giving yourself the gift of restorative sleep—one of the most powerful tools for a healthy and fulfilling life.

Here's to peaceful nights, energized mornings, and the boundless potential that comes from a well-rested you. Sweet dreams and happy cooking!

Special Bonus: A Gift of Flavor, Health, and Vitality

Congratulations on embarking on this exciting journey with our cookbook! As a token of our appreciation for being part of our culinary and wellness community, we're thrilled to share something extra with you. In addition to the delicious recipes and expert guidance in this book, you'll gain access to five exclusive bonus resources to enhance your experience.

Your Exclusive Bonuses Include:

4 Additional Recipe Books:

Expand your collection with these inspiring cookbooks filled with a variety of meals, desserts, and snacks. From beloved classics to innovative new dishes, you'll now have a total of **300** recipes to explore, enjoy, and share.

These thoughtfully curated bonuses are designed to support your well-being, bringing balance, nourishment, and joy to your daily routine. Whether you're trying new recipes or focusing on your health goals, these resources will guide and empower you every step of the way.

How to Access Your Bonus eBooks:

1. Scan the QR Code provided.
2. Enter **$0** as the price.
3. Tap or click **"I want this."**
4. Scroll down and input your email address.
5. Enter **$0** again where it says **"Add a tip."**
6. Tap or click **"Get."**
7. Select **"Download"** or **"Send to Kindle."**

First Book

LONGEVITY DIET COOKBOOK

Longevity Diet Cookbook: Nourish Your Body for a Longer, Healthier Life

Discover the secrets to a longer, healthier life with the Longevity Diet Cookbook—your ultimate guide to eating for vitality, disease prevention, and sustained energy. Packed with nutrient-rich, anti-aging recipes, this book blends science-backed nutrition with delicious meals designed to enhance longevity, boost immunity, and promote overall well-being. From superfood-packed breakfasts to wholesome dinners and rejuvenating teas, every recipe is crafted to support cellular health, brain function, heart wellness, and gut balance. Whether you're looking to prevent chronic diseases, improve energy levels, or simply age gracefully, this cookbook provides the tools you need to thrive at every stage of life.

Start your journey toward lifelong wellness—one delicious meal at a time!

Second Book

ANTI INFLAMMATORY COOKBBOK

Anti-Inflammatory Cookbook: Nourish Your Body, Reduce Inflammation, and Thrive

Discover the healing power of food with the Anti-Inflammatory Cookbook—your ultimate guide to reducing inflammation, boosting energy, and reclaiming your health. Packed with nutrient-dense, delicious recipes, easy-to-follow meal plans, and expert tips on lifestyle changes, this cookbook makes it simple to embrace an anti-inflammatory diet. Whether you're looking to manage chronic pain, improve digestion, or simply feel your best, these wholesome meals will help you fuel your body and fight inflammation—one bite at a time.

Third Book

HERBAL TEA REMEDIES

Herbal Tea Remedies is your ultimate guide to harnessing the healing power of nature through the art of herbal tea. Packed with time-tested wisdom, soothing recipes, and expert insights, this book explores how herbal teas can naturally boost immunity, aid digestion, relieve stress, enhance sleep, support heart health, and detoxify the body. Whether you're a tea enthusiast or new to herbal remedies, this book will help you craft delicious, therapeutic blends to nurture your body and mind—one sip at a time.

Fourth Book

IMMUNE BOOSTING SMOOTHIES AND JUICES

"Immune Boosting Smoothies and Juices" is your ultimate guide to strengthening your body's natural defenses with delicious, nutrient-packed drinks. This book features a variety of immune-supporting smoothies, detox juices, and wellness shots made with powerful superfoods like citrus fruits, leafy greens, berries, and anti-inflammatory spices. Whether you're looking to energize your mornings, support overall health, or fight off seasonal illnesses, these easy-to-make recipes will help you stay strong, vibrant, and resilient. Take control of your well-being—one sip at a time!

Made in United States
Troutdale, OR
06/16/2025

32174095R00058